Anxiety & Diet

Recipes and Foods for Ending Stress and Mood Swings

By

Michele L. McCurdy

MICHELE L. MCCURDY

Anxiety & Diet

Copyright © 2019

All rights reserved. This book or any portion thereof may not be reproduced or used in any manner whatsoever without the express written permission of the publisher except for the use of brief quotations in a book review.

ISBN: 9781697338126

Warning and Disclaimer

Every effort has been made to make this book as accurate as possible. However, no warranty or fitness is implied. The information provided is on an "as-is" basis. The author and the publisher shall have no liability or responsibility to any person or entity with respect to any loss or damages that arise from the information in this book.

MEDICAL DISCLAIMER: I am not a medical doctor and I do not advice that you stop cancer treatment to pursue an alkaline diet. The information available in this book is from my own personal research and it has not been endorsed by the medical field.

Publisher contact

Skinny Bottle Publishing

books@skinnybottle.com

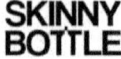

About the Author vii
    Michele L. McCurdy vii
Introduction 9
What Is Anxiety? 11
Brief History of Anxiety.. 14
Types of Anxiety.. 16
Structures of the Brain Involved in Anxiety 20
Neurotransmitters That Play A Role In Anxiety 22
Traditional Methods of Treating Anxiety Disorders....... 25
    Medications 25
    Therapy to Reduce Anxiety...................................... 27
    Other Natural Techniques to Reduce Anxiety 28
Reduce Anxiety With Diet 33
    Inflammation in the Diet... 35
Foods, Food Products and Other Substances To Avoid 43
    Caffeine.. 43
    Sugar.. 44
    Fats... 45
    Artificial Sweeteners 45
    Artificial Food Flavors... 46
    Artificial Food Colors.. 46
    Processed, Prepackaged Foods 47
    Dairy Products... 48

Preservatives 49

Gluten 50

Alcohol 51

Drugs 52

Vitamins and Minerals to Help Reduce Inflammation and Anxiety 54

Vitamin D 55

B Complex Vitamins 56

Other Vitamins and Minerals 58

Food and Drinks That Can Reduce Inflammation and Anxiety 61

Leafy Greens and Other Vegetables 62

Fruit 63

Nuts and Seeds 63

Nut Butters 64

Whole Grains 65

Oatmeal 65

Salmon and Tuna 65

Avocado 65

Beans and Lentils 66

Soy-Based Foods 66

Fermented Foods 67

Drinks to Help Calm Anxiety 68

Herbs and Spices 68

Dark Chocolate 69
Healthy Food Ideas 69
  Day 1 72
  Day 2 72
  Day 3 73
  Day 4 73
  Day 5 74
  Day 6 74
  Day 7 75
'Healthier' Recipe Ideas 76
  Quinoa Salad 76
  Black Bean Sweet Potato Enchiladas 78
  Easy Guacamole 80
  Chicken and Wild Rice Soup 81
  Potato Chickpea Curry 82
  Broccoli Tofu Stir Fry 84
  Layered Cornbread Taco Salad 86
  Homemade French Fries 87
  Portobello Burger 88
  Apple Crumble 89

MICHELE L. MCCURDY

About the Author

Michele L. McCurdy

I have worked in the mental healthcare field for two decades, most of this time in a supervisory role. My staff and I have seen amazing results when the clients we work with have improved their way of eating. By following the general guidelines described in this book, our clients have been able to lose weight, have kept it off and have improved certain health conditions. Some of them have even been able to reduce or discontinue some of their prescribed pharmaceutical medications with the guidance of their physician due to eating a better diet.

My staff and I work with our clients to adopt nutritious and tasty meal plans and weekly menus by following their specific physician and dietician recommendations. We have been able to tailor each person's meal plan for each of their health and dietary needs. This includes implementing diets that involve eating according to specific daily caloric intake (for example 1500 or 1800 calories per day). We also aim to limit sugar, saturated fats, refined carbohydrates, highly processed foods, and fatty animal products from their diets. We have been able to help our clients to increase their consumption of fresh fruits and vegetables, whole grains and nuts. Many have increased the amount of water they drink. And some have switched over to non-dairy milk. Most have greatly reduced meals out at Fast Food restaurants, in favor of healthier restaurants or home-cooked meals made by our staff.

Although I only have a degree in Psychology, I have taken University courses in Nursing, Anatomy & Physiology and Nutrition to add to my knowledge of healthy nutrition. My hobby of researching optimum diets through research-based studies has added to my knowledge base and conversation about what may be the best food to eat for certain conditions. I tend to not adhere to fad-based diets and would rather base my research on studies that have shown to improve health for the long-term. I believe that eating a balanced diet with a wide variety of whole foods helps to maintain good health or attain better health for the average person and the people I serve. I would hope that you would also be able to achieve great mental and physical health from eating better!

Introduction

Millions of people deal with anxiety every day. Anxiety can occur in the young or old, male or female. The fear that anxiety creates in a person's mind can manifest in many different physical and emotional symptoms. It can strike in any place or situation a person might be in at the time. Anxiety has a way of pervading all areas of life for certain individuals, at any given time.

An individual experiencing anxiety might have a feeling of dread or impending doom about an upcoming event of the current day or of an approaching date. Anxiety can permeate all the thoughts a person has leading up to the feared situation. It can be the first thought of the morning when a person wakes up, to the last thought a person has before they go to sleep.

Anxiety could be a fear about public speaking at school or work, or performance and test anxiety on the job or at school. Some people with anxiety are afraid to try new experiences or put themselves in new situations. These situations and many more can all cause mild to severe anxiety.

 Mild forms can include the feeling of general nervousness or unease about a situation. On the other end of the spectrum, the most severe forms of anxiety can lead to debilitating panic attacks and avoidance of specific places, people or events.

Many people wonder what they can do to ease the feeling of constant worry and dread that is experienced every so often or day after day. Many people have found, either on their own or through the guidance of their physician, mental health professional or dietician that one of the most important lifestyle changes a person can make is to eat a healthy diet. Many people from all walks of life have found a healthy diet can decrease anxiety and promote feelings of well-being in the mind and body. This includes eating a wide variety of rich, natural foods that are high in antioxidants, vitamins, minerals, and essential amino acids.

What a person eats can positively impact the functioning of the entire mind and body. To get started on this journey of healthy eating to overcome anxiety, a general overview of what anxiety is and does in people that experience it will be explained. This book will guide readers to the kinds of foods, vitamins, and minerals they can eat to reduce feelings of anxiety. Some vitamins and minerals that help combat anxiety and meal plan ideas will be included to get you started on your way!

What Is Anxiety?

Anxiety affects people of all ages, from young children to the elderly, and can occur in males and females alike. Females are more commonly affected. For some, it is a lifelong struggle that occurs on a regular basis. For others, it will come and go temporarily, depending on the situation or experience.

At some point, most people experience some form of anxiety in their life and this is normal. It can be an emotional or physical symptom that is the result of internal thoughts of stress that can be mild or intense. It is a way our mind protects ourselves from adverse or uncomfortable situations.

Anxiety is the unique way our mind helps us make important, quick decisions in times of stress. These stressful thoughts about a situation may only be perceived by the mind and may not pose a physical threat to our safety and well-being. Anxiety can also strike in a situation where we are truly facing some difficult obstacles or real physical danger.

There are some thoughts and feelings that a person who experiences anxiety might be feeling. The human body has a unique way of letting us know when real or perceived danger might be imminent. A person worrying about something may feel a wide range of emotions during times of stress. It might be trepidation, fear, terror, helplessness, loss of control, irritation, agitation and a general sense of uneasiness in one or more areas of life. Sometimes these emotions manifest unexpectedly in other areas of life that don't even seem to be related to the stressor that is causing the anxiety.

More physical effects like nausea and even vomiting can occur, too. Skin conditions such as hives or eczema can manifest.

When anxiety occurs, some people may experience intense physical reactions to perceived fear or real danger that they might not have felt before or that occurs each time anxiety strikes. Each person experiences anxiety differently. Some might have one or two symptoms caused by stress, another person might have many of them.

The symptoms of anxiety cause one or more physical symptoms such as mild or profuse sweating, blushing, hot flashes or feeling faint. In extreme cases, a person may even pass out or briefly lose consciousness. Nausea and even vomiting can occur. As anxiety rises so does blood pressure. Some people feel their heart pounding or racing, have shortness of breath, and even physical pain in different areas of the body. Muscles can become tense and cannot easily be relaxed. A person may find they are so anxious they temporarily lose the ability to speak or are unable to speak clearly or in whole sentences. In some situations, a person may feel the inability to think clearly as if every thought in the mind disappears for a brief moment or longer.

It can be momentarily crippling when one or more of these symptoms of anxiety is experienced, either unexpectedly or in anticipation of it. Anxiety can cause a mild or extreme physical reaction to events in life that might be totally safe (just not perceived this way) or verifiably terrifying and dangerous. It is the human body's way of keeping safe, of ultimate self-preservation.

Anxiety is the mind and body's way of processing and dealing with stress in uncomfortable or new, unfamiliar situations. It can also be a reaction to intense internal stressors that can occur in everyday life. Anxiety can also occur when extreme danger to normal, common, everyday life experiences are perceived in the mind to be life-threatening or dangerous in some terrible, uncompromising way.

Brief History of Anxiety

In early humans, there were many possibilities for natural events to occur that could potentially cause fear and anxiety. This reaction would be a cause for a person to make a life-saving decision in a split second. A dangerous natural event such as a flash flood or an encounter with a wild, aggressive animal of large size might be cause for action. A human in this situation, present or past, would feel the need for immediate action.

In the case of a flash flood, for example, a person would realize the need to run to safety immediately. It would be a cause to flee. In the other case, it could be to flee or fight. This "Fight or Flight" reaction is understood as a plausible cause for an individual to react swiftly and with fear.

In modern times, humans have a reaction to what is perceived in the mind to be a terrible, threatening, dangerous or uncomfortable situation and it is called anxiety. For some individuals, anxiety can cause the same reaction as it did for early humans. The need for "Fight or

Flight" is still a common means to achieve a safe, calm and comfortable state of mind.

When facing an anxiety-provoking situation, there are some individuals who might have no feeling of fear at all. For others, mild to severe forms of anxiety along with related symptoms can result in a varied range of physical and/or emotional reactions.

A person who experiences mild anxiety may be able to deal with the feelings and reactions calmly. For example, anxiety can be caused by giving a speech in front of classmates in the classroom. No one may even notice the anxiety being experienced. Another person might blush and start sweating when talking in front of the class. For yet another, the same situation could result in a magnified feeling of terror and loss of control, even though there may not be a physical danger. Sometimes the thoughts and feelings can be so intense the person needs to leave the situation, so the anxiety can subside. In the extreme case, this would be the "Flight" aspect of anxiety; fleeing the situation to make the uncomfortable feelings go away. Everyone experiences anxiety differently.

Types of Anxiety

People can experience many different types of anxiety. A person may experience one type or more than one at the same time. For the purpose of focusing more on a diet that helps reduce anxiety, a general overview of the types of anxiety that exist will be reviewed. The purpose of this book is to help those that may already know they have anxiety and to find out ways to decrease these feelings with diet.

Generalized Anxiety Disorder or (GAD) is characterized by constant worry on most days for a period of six months or more. The persistent worry generally can be unrealistic and occurs across all areas of life. This can include worrying about relationships, money, work or school. It usually affects the ability to live day-to-day life normally. Normal daily tasks may seem overwhelming. This amount of worry is what sets people apart from the average person that worries from time to time about things. Friends and family may not even know a person is suffering from GAD. The person may appear to be acting and doing things normally, or even overachieving in life.

Underneath the calm façade, a person may be suffering from constant worry.

Social Anxiety Disorder or Social Phobia is experienced when a person has a fear of being in social situations. This affects their ability to act or feel normally in a situation that involves other people. It can be in a specific social setting, such as with a group of friends or in a public place such as a restaurant or in school. Many people that experience social anxiety disorder suffer from it starting at a young age. The person may enjoy having close friends and other people in their lives, but they have a limit on how much time with others they can tolerate before the anxiety gets too high.

Agoraphobia is the fear of people. A person experiencing agoraphobia can be afraid of being in or around groups of people. Situations like the school setting, concerts, public places, sports venues, restaurants, parties and other areas where large groups of people congregate can cause anxiety to manifest. People who experience this tend to avoid places where there are lots of people.

Panic Disorder is dominated by one or more acute episodes of panic attacks. A panic attack can be described as an intense emotional and physical response to anxiety triggered by a very stressful thought or situation. This can either happen when a person experiences familiar stressors and triggers or may occur suddenly when least expected. Not all people that suffer from anxiety experience panic attacks. Having a panic attack can affect a person's ability to experience a situation normally in a calm way and can be very disrupting, upsetting and embarrassing. The Fight or Flight response is heightened and the person experiencing it may need to get away from the situation immediately to take time alone to calm down.

Obsessive-Compulsive Disorder (OCD) is an anxiety disorder that occurs when a person has repeated thoughts or actions that they cannot stop. These can occur multiple times in a day and can be pervasive affecting all areas of life. A person cannot seem to shake the same thoughts or actions from happening, even though they are aware they should stop. OCD behavior can have a profoundly negative effect on daily life and interrupts normal functioning.

Post-Traumatic Stress Disorder (PTSD) is an anxiety disorder that develops when a person has experienced a previous traumatic event. PTSD can be caused when a person has experienced a natural disaster, accident or other extreme or violent event. A person develops increasing anxiety from the inability to stop reliving or experiencing the event in the mind. The same intense emotions that the person experienced at the time of the event can resurface causing the person to experience or replay the event over and over. A person living with PTSD may have nightmares or hallucinations in reaction to the traumatic event. This can last for a very long time without effective treatment. It can very negatively affect the quality of life for someone that has PTSD. Many common feelings experienced when someone has PTSD include irritability, anger, hallucinations, trembling, sweating and the need to avoid situations that may trigger anxiety.

There are also many other types of phobias that people experience that may be specific to each person. Many people have anxiety or fear of specific situations or objects they encounter in their life. The anxiety that occurs because of the phobia that a person has can be mild to severe. Phobias that people have can be as varied as each individual is. Some examples of phobias that people have are the fear of snakes, spiders, dirt or uncleanliness, ticks, cockroaches, elevators, heights, being in enclosed spaces, deep water, eating in the presence of others or performance anxiety. These are just some examples of the types of fear that some people have. A person can have a phobia about any object, experience or situation that can affect living life normally.

Structures of the Brain Involved in Anxiety

The limbic system is a part of the brain that plays a major role in the chemical processes and relay of messages associated with anxiety. It consists of the amygdala, hippocampus, hypothalamus, and thalamus which are all in the same area of the brain. Scientists are still learning about the complex role these parts of the brain play in anxiety. These structures are located deep inside the brain. The parts of the limbic system communicate when a person is having anxiety.

The amygdala is the active area of the brain where emotions like fear and anger develop. In people suffering from anxiety, this area of the brain is often overactive. Brain scans using functional magnetic resonance imaging (also referred to as fMRI) and PET scans show certain areas of the brain, such as the amygdala, that show active neuronal activity when a person is experiencing anxiety.

The hippocampus is the area of the brain involved in memory retention. In the case of anxiety, memories are made that involve fear. When these memories are triggered, it sends a message to the amygdala to activate the fear response.

The hypothalamus is the part of the limbic system that sends and receives messages to and from the amygdala. The area of the brain called the thalamus also plays a role in anxiety. The amygdala sends messages to the thalamus when a person is under stress or anxiety. These messages result in the release of certain brain chemicals that activate a response in the body to anxiety.

Neurotransmitters That Play A Role In Anxiety

To better understand what is happening when an individual is experiencing anxiety, doctors and other researchers have taken a better look at what is happening from a scientific perspective. There are many complex chemical processes in the brain that occur when a person is experiencing anxiety. The neurotransmitters are the chemical messengers in the brain that send messages between the brain cells. They act in the synapses, or gaps, between the brain cells to increase or decrease the experience of anxiety. Neurotransmitters are released and then are absorbed by neighboring brain cells, in different amounts, depending on what is needed and available by the brain.

Serotonin, GABA, dopamine, tryptophan, norepinephrine, epinephrine and cortisol are some of the neurotransmitters that play a major role in causing the feeling of anxiety. Some of these can be found to be too low or too high in the brain or body. They all act in different ways with each other but are very important. Eating foods that contain an adequate level of essential vitamins, minerals, and amino acids can affect the amount of these neurotransmitters in the brain. If any of these are deficient, it can affect a person's mood and increase feelings of anxiety. A quick explanation of each of these will be explored.

Serotonin is the key neurotransmitter that plays an active role in the brain cells to increase or decrease anxiety levels. It is sometimes known as the 'happy' chemical of the brain. It contributes to feelings of well-being and comfort. Having an inadequate serotonin level in the brain cells can increase feelings of anxiousness.

GABA (or gamma-aminobutyric acid) is also a neurotransmitter that plays an important role in anxiety. GABA is the calming or inhibitory transmitter. It is found to be low in people that have anxiety. It is important to keep GABA at the appropriate level in the brain to control excitatory feelings. Serotonin balances out the effects of GABA in the brain resulting in a better mood and less anxiety.

Tryptophan and dopamine are two other neurotransmitters that help play a role in balancing mood. Dopamine can either act as an inhibitory or excitatory transmitter. Appropriate levels of these chemicals in the brain help a person feel calm and experience less anxiety. They also help to provide better sleep, a more balanced mood and can increase motivation.

Norepinephrine and epinephrine are the excitatory neurotransmitters of the brain. Norepinephrine can also be found in the bloodstream when the adrenal glands in the body release it. When these chemicals are released, this results in a high level of adrenaline in the body. This is important during times of stress and anxiety to mobilize or cause the person to react to danger or perceived danger. On the other hand, when there is a high level of norepinephrine and epinephrine, a person will feel jittery or nervous, have an increased heart rate and quick, shallow breathing. A person will experience feelings that are similar to panic or high anxiety when there is a high level of these excitatory neurotransmitters in the body.

Cortisol is a lot like norepinephrine and epinephrine in the way that it acts in the body. It is the body's stress hormone that increases when a person is under stress or anxiety. Too much cortisol in the body system over long periods of time can lead to negative health effects. It can contribute to inflammatory responses in the body that may lead to diseases like high blood pressure, cancer, and diabetes. It can also make a person's immune system weak and the person will get sick more often. When cortisol is too high the body is working overtime trying to bring cortisol down to normal levels. This places great stress on the body's systems resulting in the inflammatory response.

Traditional Methods of Treating Anxiety Disorders

Medications

Physicians and psychiatrists regularly turn to a few major types of medications to help treat anxiety. Different medications work better for different people. Some medications do not work well at all for some people. These medications attempt to treat the symptoms of anxiety but do not help solve the root issues that anxiety is caused by. Medications can provide temporary relief until the source of anxiety can be resolved.

A brief review of only some of the pharmaceutical options available will be covered. For this type of treatment, your physician or mental healthcare professional will know what is best for you to try. Sometimes a combination of medications, therapy, and diet will be the best way to combat feelings of anxiety. This will be up to you and your healthcare practitioner to decide.

Selective Serotonin Reuptake Inhibitors or SSRIs are a commonly used pharmaceutical drug used to treat anxiety. These act to prevent the uptake of serotonin into the brain cells so more is available to use. Since serotonin has a calming effect on people, when more serotonin is present, it can act to relieve anxiety. The effects of SSRIs take a couple to a few weeks to start working fully for an individual. They may not work for everyone or may lessen anxiety only minimally. As with all medications, dosages may need to be increased or decreased after the person has been taking it for a few weeks to try to maximize effectiveness.

Selective Serotonin Norepinephrine Inhibitors or SSNIs also act to prevent brain cell uptake of serotonin. In addition, they inhibit the hormone norepinephrine from being released into the body. Higher norepinephrine levels can be excitatory and stimulate the anxiety response in a person. Keeping the norepinephrine levels low can be helpful to keep the anxiety response low.

Benzodiazepines have an inhibitory effect on the central nervous system. These types of medications have a relaxing or sedative effect on the body. This type of medication can be used short-term for quick effectiveness, such as during an acute episode of heightened anxiety or for panic attacks.

As with all pharmaceutical drugs, they have the risk of unwanted side effects. Using benzodiazepines can cause dependence if used regularly, so they are not recommended for long-term use. The sedative effects can prevent a person from doing everyday activities.

Drowsiness is a common side effect. Effectiveness will decrease over time unless the dosage is increased. If possible, it is best to find other methods to relieve anxiety that do not involve long-term use of this drug.

Therapy to Reduce Anxiety

Psychotherapy or 'talking therapy' is the traditional approach to getting a handle on the mental issues that people experience. This applies to treating symptoms of anxiety as well. Psychotherapy can be a good way to investigate what is causing anxiety for someone. It can be therapeutic for a person to talk about how the anxiety affecting their day to day activities. Although much can be uncovered when finding out 'why' a person has anxiety, there is another method to treat anxiety that seems to be more effective at treating symptoms.

This is Cognitive Behavior Therapy, otherwise known as CBT. Cognitive Behavior Therapy is the standard method for treating anxiety disorders and is quite helpful. CBT has been found to be one of the most effective ways to deal with anxiety, in addition to adding healthy daily routines like eating right and exercising. Sometimes, CBT is used in conjunction with pharmaceutical medication to increase success in treatment.

Cognitive behavior therapy includes working with a therapist to develop and practice coping methods to deal with anxiety. It includes practicing techniques and exercises for the person to use to prevent anxiety or panic attacks from occurring or while experiencing anxiety. Often, CBT includes replaying in the mind or re-creating an anxiety-provoking situation in the company of the therapist. When anxiety is triggered, the therapist will be able to teach effective methods to cope with the situation that the person can use on their own in everyday life.

For example, if a person has a fear of taking an elevator, the therapist will work with the person practicing steps to slowly become more comfortable doing this. This usually takes a large time commitment but is very effective. A person and the therapist may start the therapy talking about elevators until the fear subsides. The next step may be talking together outside of an elevator. When that fear has been dealt with, the person and therapist will try stepping into the elevator. The therapist will work with the person at each step until their anxiety subsides. The main goal will be to inch closer to the feared event or situation while learning coping mechanisms as anxiety rises. The final goal will be for the person to practice doing the feared activity or being in the feared situation with the company and support of the therapist. This seems to be very effective for a person that is determined to conquer their fear.

Other Natural Techniques to Reduce Anxiety

There are certainly other ways of treating anxiety aside from pharmaceutical drugs. A person can work on reducing anxiety by adopting a healthy diet and by making other better lifestyle choices. Doing these two things can be more effective than taking pharmaceuticals, for some people. If you and your doctor have determined that pharmaceutical drugs are still necessary, to some extent, there are still activities to incorporate into daily life that can lessen the feeling of anxiety.

By keeping busy and incorporating some healthy lifestyle activities like these into daily life, there will be less time to worry and more outlets to diffuse the nervous energy that anxiety creates.

To work at reducing anxiety, some of these lifestyle choices can be done as a daily routine. They can also be done intermittently when there is time or when necessary. There are many more activities and ideas based on interests and abilities, but some of these include:

> 30 minutes of daily exercise – Everyone can benefit by incorporating exercise into their day. Endorphins, the 'feel-good' hormones, are released into the bloodstream after exercise. This naturally helps to reduce anxiety. Taking a walk, hiking, bike riding, swimming, and jogging are all easy free ways to get some exercise into your daily routine immediately. If the option exists, take the stairs at work and anywhere else there is the choice between the elevator or stairs (doctor's offices, apartment buildings, shopping malls, etc.). At the grocery store or mall, park as far away as you can and use that as a short walk to get your daily exercise in small increments.

> Join a health club, an exercise group or take a specific exercise class. This could be something that has always interested you, such as yoga, pilates, spinning, dance, swimming or your local walking, biking or running club. Many areas, even in small

towns, have groups that get together to get people moving and stay physically active at least once per week. There are endless groups on social media to join for motivation and ideas to get a person up and exercising.

Create an active social life as an outlet to reduce anxiety. A person should seek out and develop and maintain an active social life at all stages of life. Sometimes this can be difficult when moving to a new city full of strangers, starting a new job or a when person is in a new phase of life (such as graduating from school or being a new mother). Studies have shown that people live longer, have less anxiety and are generally happier when they are able to maintain a strong social network. This network can consist of family, friends, neighbors, coworkers, and acquaintances. These provide more outlets for people they can talk to and do activities with on a regular basis.

To get started, join a club or take a class where you can find others that share your interests (gardening club, chess club, book club, lunch club are examples). Some people find that going to church and participating in associated smaller groups within their church provides ample opportunity to engage in an active social life.

Volunteering at a favorite organization can help increase social interactions and provide another social outlet. A person should participate in a volunteer opportunity to see if they will enjoy it.

Sometimes it takes finding the right organization that fits a person's temperament and interests. Volunteering can provide great satisfaction and add fulfillment to a person's life. There are places that people are usually easily able to volunteer at that include a local homeless shelter, food bank, political organization or non-profit group.

Working actively to reduce daily stress by other natural methods can also reduce anxiety. Some people incorporate daily meditation, or schedule weekly or monthly massages to reduce stress. Sometimes taking a few minutes out of each day to practice slow, calming breathing helps to relieve anxiety. Many people find that the addition of scent aromatherapy in their home or work environment using candles or essential oils can be very helpful. Some find regular chiropractic care or acupuncture treatments when anxiety is high or to prevent it from getting worse, can effectively reduce anxiety. For others, taking time out to listen to some favorite music, see a live band or concert or play an instrument is effective. For more artistic types of people, distracting the mind with activities like painting, drawing or writing in a journal will help calm the nerves. There are also many interesting adult coloring books available to buy that many people find calming.

A person should make sure to get enough sleep. For most people to function effectively, 7 or 8 hours of sleep per night is recommended. Some people can get by on a little less, and some feel a little more sleep is better for them. When a person does not get adequate rest, some symptoms similar to anxiety can occur. Inability to focus, restlessness, irritability and mood changes can happen. Being fatigued can also make current levels of anxiety worsen. It is sometimes very helpful to incorporate a short nap into each day to help calm the nerves. Anxiety can be very tiring when the mind is on constant alert or in a hypervigilant state of worry.

By keeping the mind distracted and not focused on the stress or stressors, this will lessen anxiety for at least a short period of time and will be beneficial to the whole body. It is very important for a person experiencing anxiety to reduce stress from work, family or other outside influences. Incorporating all of these lifestyle choices and choosing to eat a healthier diet will help a person suffering from anxiety to feeling better.

Reduce Anxiety With Diet

By choosing to take an active role in reducing anxiety in all areas of life, there is one crucial area that should not be ignored. Eating a healthy diet is a major factor to consider when trying to reduce anxiety. For some people, making the change to eat healthily can be a very difficult lifestyle adjustment. Others may already be on their path to healthier eating for a variety of other personal or health reasons. For some, just getting to experience a life of reduced anxiety is a profound benefit that encourages someone to maintain a healthy diet.

A person suffering from anxiety can also experience improved mood by maintaining healthy body weight. Sometimes a person struggling with their weight (whether too high or too low) can have feelings of low self-confidence, lack of motivation and being self-conscious, which heightens anxiety. This anxiety can be lessened by eating a healthy, low-fat diet full of fresh, nutritional foods. By being able to attain a weight that is recommended for gender, build, age and height, a person will be able to experience good mental health that includes less anxiety.

A good place to start eating healthy to reduce anxiety is by following the recommended daily servings of fruits and vegetables. For the average 2000 calorie per day diet, there are general recommendations of amounts of foods for people to eat each day. There are many websites with calculators to determine specific amounts for each person to eat depending on their age, height, weight, and gender.

In general, an average adult should eat at least 2-4 servings of fruits, 5-7 servings of vegetables, 5 ounces of protein, 6 ounces of whole grains and 3 cups of dairy per day (other options exist for those on a whole-food, plant-based diet). These will vary depending on dietary needs and preferences. Each person should research what amount is best for them to eat. Depending on other dietary and health needs, a person should meet with a dietician or other health professional for specific recommendations.

 A good area to focus on when trying to maintain or achieve a healthy weight is the BMI or Body Mass Index calculator. The BMI is a formula of height and weight that measures body fat. Health professionals use this to determine what a healthy weight an individual should be. This number will also be a goal to aim for when trying to lose weight.

Many websites offer a free online calculator to determine this number easily. It can also be found by following this formula: weight in pounds, divided by height in inches, squared, multiplied by 703.

For example, for someone that weighs 150 pounds and is 5 feet, 6 inches tall, the formula would be 150 divided by (66 x 66 = 4,356) x 703. 150 divided by 4,356 = 0.03443526170798 x 703 = 24.2 (rounded). Use this number, 24.2, to find out body mass index, which will indicate if this person is at a healthy weight. By looking at the chart below, we find that the person is within a normal BMI range and weight.

Underweight = less than 18.5

Normal weight = 18.5 – 24.9

Overweight = 25 – 29.9

Obese = 30 or greater

By following the recommended BMI scale, a person will be well on their way to reducing extra body weight and feeling great physically. This will positively affect feelings of overall good mental health and well-being and therefore can reduce feelings of anxiety.

Inflammation in the Diet

When eating a diet that helps reduce anxiety, it is very important to understand how inflammation from the foods that are eaten plays a role. Inflammation in the body can cause a whole host of health issues. If there is a genetic component to anxiety, inflammation can trigger the genes that cause anxiety in some people. If inflammation occurs for an extended amount of time, larger and more serious health problems manifest.

Inflammation is the human body's way of dealing with the onslaught of unhealthy threats the body is exposed to each day. Toxins from the foods we eat, pollution in the environment or stress and anxiety all contribute to inflammation. The entire immune system reacts to reduce or prevent the buildup of toxins in the body to maintain good health and ward off disease. Reducing the level of inflammation in the body can go a long way to lessen anxiety. By lessening inflammation from occurring, the body will have fewer defenses engaged in trying to maintain optimal body function.

The modern diet that most people eat today seems to include a whole host of foods that cause inflammation and health issues in the body. This is sometimes referred to as the Standard Western Diet or Standard American Diet (SAD). This diet has shown to increase the number of people that experience mental health issues and physical problems. Chronic diseases like high cholesterol, heart disease, diabetes, obesity, and cancer have become commonplace in developed countries because of this way of eating. People that eat the Standard Western Diet consume many processed foods. This diet is typically high in saturated fat, cholesterol, sodium, and sugar. It doesn't take a doctor or scientist to realize that this way of eating is not healthy.

The inflammation caused by eating unhealthy food can lead to heightened anxiety. This forces the body to work overtime to balance and maintain homeostasis, which is our body's way of functioning at an optimum level. With inflammation in the body, a person can develop high blood sugar, high blood pressure, high cholesterol, brain fog, and numerous bodily aches and pains and health ailments. It is smart to try and reduce inflammation in the body to reduce feelings of anxiety.

Feelings of general anxiety can come from not feeling healthy overall because of bad diet. It can also come from having to deal with and treat the multitude of chronic health issues or diseases, caused by this diet. This can mean frequent monitoring by health professionals resulting in many doctor appointments and may require taking daily medications. This causes many people to worry about the cost of the treatments and medications or worrying about overall general health. By taking small steps to improve diet, this will help reduce anxiety caused by the repercussions of inflammation in the body.

People that suffer from food allergies can suffer from anxiety as well. If allergies are undiagnosed, the foods eaten can cause inflammation throughout the entire body. It is said that most of the serotonin produced in the body is in the gut and intestines. Serotonin levels in the brain can be altered, resulting in anxiety and other mental health issues. It is important to be aware that what is eaten might be causing low serotonin levels and to be tested for food allergies if this seems to be a problem. There is still much research to be done on this, but worth taking note to follow future advancements and discoveries in this area.

Inflammation in the body can also be caused by toxins from pesticides and herbicides from the foods we eat. As a general rule, it is most helpful if a person can avoid foods sprayed by these types of chemicals whenever possible. There can be numerous chemicals on fruits and vegetables from farming techniques using herbicides and pesticides. They are left in small and large amounts on food and cannot always be washed off.

If possible, find local farmers that use organic food farming methods to purchase food. Certain nutrient levels and the quality of food is increased when it is grown local and organic. It can be immensely helpful to contact the company or talk to the grower or producer of your food. It is important to know where your food is grown and will help to ensure the farming methods used are safe for you and the environment. Since this type of food is not shipped long distances, it is usually grown in-season and picked when ripe. It will be the freshest and will have a better overall taste, too. Reducing the consumption of chemicals through the diet this way has shown to be beneficial for mental and physical health and will reduce bodily inflammation.

Many cities have Farmer's Markets where fresh, high-quality locally grown food can be purchased. Buying from a Farmer's Market is a really easy way to find out where your food comes from and if it contains any pesticides or herbicides. Sometimes being able to access healthy, local food is cost-prohibitive. A person might not live anywhere near a Farmer's Market or other local growers in their area. Just do the best to find high-quality, organic food that is in its natural state. If not, be sure to read food labels to determine if any chemicals have been added. Try to limit purchasing processed and pre-packaged food since those usually contain more added chemicals that promote inflammation.

Another option for some people is to grow as much of your own food as possible. For some, starting a garden is feasible and can produce more than enough healthy produce. Imagine the foods that are found in backyard gardens. Most people do not use harmful chemicals to help their gardens flourish. Fresh carrots, peas, strawberries, rhubarb, raspberries, squash, broccoli, lettuce, green beans are usually easy to grow without the use of herbicides and pesticides. These are the foods people should be eating for optimal health and feelings of mental well-being, which will reduce anxiety.

For others, who may not have a yard, some foods and herbs can be grown indoors and do well. Another option is finding a community garden. Some cities and towns have community gardens where a small plot of land can be used for individuals to plant, cultivate and harvest fruits and vegetables. With some creativity, there are many options to attain at least a fair amount of healthy, fresh food that is not sprayed with pesticides and herbicides.

Another effective way that some people find very effective at reducing inflammation that comes from the diet is to eat a vegetarian, vegan or a whole-food, plant-based diet. The attention to research by scientists and doctors to the health benefits that come from these diets seem to be increasing every day. There are many stories of people who have completely changed their physical and mental health for the better by adopting a diet that is primarily plant-based. This way of eating does not include meat, dairy and vegetable oils or limits the consumption of them. It focuses on natural, unprocessed foods like fruits, vegetables, nuts, and seeds.

There are entire groups of people and physicians on social media and blogs that aim to teach others how to reach optimal physical and mental health by following a whole-food, plant-based diet. It is easy to join some of these groups to gain ideas, recipes, and support to maintain healthy eating. Many top athletes around the world have adopted a plant-based diet with great and continued success in their sport.

Probiotics are a very important tool to help to reduce inflammation in the body. They can be added to the daily diet to preserve or enhance the normal stomach and gut bacteria. The stomach and gut contain millions of healthy bacteria or microorganisms. They are essential to keeping the whole body healthy and operating normally.

If the balance of those healthy bacteria is altered, brain health and functioning can result in mood changes such as anxiety. The immune system can also be negatively affected which causes the body to work harder to stay healthy. These beneficial gut bacteria can be destroyed by eating an unhealthy diet full of processed foods. In addition, chemical additives, antibiotics, and stress are also detrimental and cause inflammation. A healthy gut needs adequate amounts of the right kinds of bacteria for the body to function at an optimum level.

As more research has become available, it is apparent that inflammation can cause a whole host of health issues in the human body. A poor diet not only can contribute to anxiety, but other health issues will become apparent over time. Health problems such as high blood pressure, obesity, heart disease, arthritis, dementia, diabetes, fibromyalgia are just some examples of problems caused by eating an unhealthy diet. Other mental health problems may occur, too, such as depression and ADHD.

It is worth mentioning that diabetes is now a common disease that is caused by eating an unhealthy modern diet. It causes many problems throughout the body and affects many different systems as it progresses. It can have negative effects on the eyes, kidneys, circulation, nerves, heart and more. The symptoms and some of the health problems associated with Type 2 diabetes can be lessened by eating a wholesome, nutrient-dense diet.

Diabetes results when the body can no longer effectively process sugar in the blood. The pancreas acts to help process the sugar that comes into the body from the diet. As high amounts of sugar and products containing sugar are consumed, it needs to be processed and broken down. The pancreas works harder and harder to break this sugar down. As time progresses, the pancreas is not able to do an effective job of breaking sugar down and excreting it from the body. This can result in extremely high or low levels of sugar in the blood. The level of blood sugar will fluctuate depending on what the person eats. These swings in blood sugar result in some of the same symptoms that people with anxiety suffer such as nervousness, trembling, rapid heartbeat and excessive sweating.

Foods, Food Products and Other Substances To Avoid

The following foods, drinks or ingredients that are added to many foods may cause symptoms of anxiety and are important to become more knowledgeable about. There are many reputable sources to research more details and names of items that may contain these products or ingredients. Consuming some of these products may increase the anxiety that is already occurring in some people. It is best to reduce or eliminate them from your diet, if possible.

Caffeine

Drinking caffeinated beverages like coffee and soda can produce many of the same effects as anxiety. In some individuals, unwanted physical symptoms can manifest. These can mimic what happens to a person experiencing anxiety or a panic attack. These can include increased heart rate, increased blood pressure, sweating and a pounding, racing heart. Anxiety-sufferers can usually recognize when they have consumed too much caffeine. The more caffeine that is consumed, the more heightened the feeling of anxiety gets. Once this is recognized, the person can slow, reduce or eliminate caffeine consumption altogether for the sake of not exacerbating the onset of feelings of anxiety.

Energy drinks are no better. They contain extremely high amounts of caffeine and sugar. They also have other additives and flavors that can cause an inflammatory effect on the body. The high sugar will cause blood sugar to spike. After a while, the sugar and caffeine in the blood dip down quickly producing an extreme low in energy and blood sugar. The intense fluctuation of blood sugar levels is difficult for the mind and body to adjust to.

Sugar

The typical white sugar found in the store is bleached. If you do include sweetened foods in your diet, try to find more natural, unrefined sweeteners. These can include natural unbleached cane sugar, sucanat, turbinado, honey, and agave. Use all forms of sugar sparingly, as these produce excitatory and inflammatory effects in the body. Sugar can act as a stimulant, causing increased anxiety or symptoms of anxiety like nervousness, trembling and sweating.

Highly processed sugars go by many names. It is very important to read food labels to determine if sugars are added. In many cases, more than one type of sugar is added. Other names for highly processed sugars include high fructose corn syrup, corn syrup, beet sugar, beet syrup, fructose, sucrose, dextrose, maltose, brown sugar, and rice syrup.

Fats

Highly refined fats such as margarine, butter, shortening, lard, and other oils and fats should be used minimally or avoided. Vegetable oils like coconut oil, olive oil, avocado oil, grapeseed oil, canola oil, and soybean oil are cheap and plently available but should also be limited in the diet. The Omega-6 fatty acids from these highly processed products can cause inflammation. Many people easily consume too many Omega-6 fatty acids. These oils can be from healthy plant sources but are still highly processed and can accumulate in the arteries and contribute to high cholesterol. They are also high in calories so can contribute to weight gain. Eating high levels of trans fats, saturated fats and hydrogenated fats in the diet can cause an inflammatory effect in the body and should be avoided whenever possible.

Artificial Sweeteners

Some people prefer to use artificial sweeteners thinking they are taking a healthy approach to consuming sugar-flavored foods or drinks. These products are lab-created food sweeteners approved by the government for human consumption that contain no nutritional value. Some people use them to cut down on calories, sugar, and carbohydrates in their daily diet. Many people are learning that there are many unwanted side effects on health that people may experience by using them. Many artificial sweeteners have a long list of problems associated with each of them. Some even cause symptoms that are the same as those that occur during periods of anxiety such as mood changes and panic attacks. For those that experience anxiety, it is best to avoid artificial sweeteners. Artificial sweeteners come by many names, either generic or brand name. Some of these are aspartame, Saccharin, acesulfame potassium, neotame, sucralose.

Artificial Food Flavors

A healthy diet should not include highly processed, lab-formulated artificial flavors. These usually originate from either chemical components or a combination of chemical and natural ingredients. There are hundreds of combinations of artificial flavors that are created from a multitude of different ingredients. They increase the desirable flavor, texture or appearance of food products. They contain no nutritive value. Artificial and other ingredients listed on food labels as 'natural flavors' can cause an inflammatory effect in the body. Many experience anxiety-like symptoms from these additives. Some people experience mild to severe migraine headaches, increased blood pressure, heart palpitations, dizziness, and other undesirable side effects.

Artificial Food Colors

Just a quick glance at food labels in any store will indicate that many foods have artificial colors in them. These can increase irritability and agitation which increases feelings of anxiety. In some children and even adults, exposure to artificial colors can cause hyperactivity. It is best to avoid them whenever possible. Red 40, Yellow 5, Yellow 6 and Blue 1 are some common artificial colors that are used in some foods and food products today. They are used in processed, packaged foods like soft drinks, candy, fruit snacks, condiments, desserts, and even pickles. Most artificial colorings are added to make processed food look better or more appetizing. They are also used to enhance a natural food's appearance (such as injecting meat with red dye).

Processed, Prepackaged Foods

It is best to eat food as nature intended, in its whole form, such as a real piece of fruit or vegetable. Anything in a package that is not in its natural state is most likely not good for a person to eat. The common term for this type of food is 'junk food.' They are often high in saturated fat, sodium, cholesterol, and sugar which all cause an inflammatory effect in the body. These highly-processed products include food-like items such as packaged desserts, bakery goods, candy, candy bars, potato chips, crackers, frozen meals, canned meals, breaded meats like pork, chicken strips and fish strips, deli meat, cheese, sausages, and bacon.

Most of the time, highly processed foods are cheaper to buy and more convenient. Many people find themselves eating convenience junk foods when they didn't intend to. A lot of people lead very busy lives and find they need to eat on the run. Or they get hungry while on the go so need to grab something quick and easy to eat. Processed, prepackaged foods can be found at places such as a gas station convenience store, drug store or mall food court.

Another huge culprit in causing inflammation throughout the body is eating at fast-food restaurants. Fast food is highly processed and most often contains high levels of fat, sodium, carbohydrates, sugars, synthetic preservatives, colorings, and additives. A quick look at any nutrition information document from a fast food restaurant will indicate this. Most of the drinks at fast-food restaurants are also full of sugar, artificial sweeteners, artificial colors, and artificial flavors. These include soda pop, milkshakes, specialty coffee drinks, and smoothies. These are all components added to food that most people should not eat regularly to obtain or maintain good physical or mental health.

Fast food products are designed to cook quickly and look good, but not always taste good or be healthy. The ingredients and cooking methods are streamlined at each fast food restaurant chain. The goal is for the food to look, feel and taste identical at each location. Most fast food will not be fresh, healthy food choices and are shipped thousands of miles to each restaurant. It is best to eat fast food minimally or avoid it altogether.

Dairy Products

Research studies have found that foods made with animal milk can cause inflammation for many babies, children, and adults. This predominately includes products from animal sources like cows and goats. Animal milk contains high levels of naturally-occurring maternal hormones and animal proteins that are not necessary for human survival. People can now adequately consume enough vegetables rich in calcium that calcium from animal milk is not necessary. Some people do prefer it, though.

Eating or drinking products from a nursing cow or other animal can cause a whole host of health issues for humans. Dairy products contain animal proteins casein and whey. Many people have an adverse reaction to these proteins and are lactose-intolerant. This can cause inflammation, an allergic reaction, and physical discomfort. Milk product consumption can cause hives, excessive mucus production in the throat, bloating, stomach discomfort and diarrhea. In some people, congestion, wheezing, breathing problems and anaphylactic reaction can occur. A severe reaction will require immediate medical attention.

Preservatives

Food-grade preservatives are added to processed foods to increase shelf life, prevent spoilage and improve texture and desirable flavor. The preservatives used in prepared, prepackaged meals and foods are most often artificial compounds created in a lab. They are not usually healthy for us to be consuming and can cause inflammation and anxiety-like symptoms. Some of the names of preservatives are difficult to pronounce which is an even better reason to stay away from them. If you don't know what it is, don't eat it.

Preservatives can be found in popular snack foods such as packaged desserts, crackers, potato chips, and candies. They can also be found in seasoning mixes, premade soups, sauces, cured meats, jerky, canned food, frozen meals, and condiments.

There are many widely used preservatives used today. MSG or monosodium glutamate is a popular food flavoring and preservative that can aggravate and contribute to feelings of anxiety in many people. MSG can cause headaches and symptoms of anxiety like nervousness, sweating, mood swings, and panic. Another common preservative that people are learning more about is carrageenan. It is a food additive that can cause migraines and stomach upset. It is added to food to lengthen its shelf-life by thickening and maintaining consistency. Other preservatives to be aware of are sodium nitrates and nitrites, BHA, BHT, and sodium benzoate. There are hundreds more used in common food products. Again, it is important to read food labels to see if these are being used in the foods you choose to eat.

Gluten

Some nutritional studies have shown that gluten can increase feelings of anxiety in people that are gluten-intolerant. Gluten is found in food or food products that contain any sort of wheat, barley or rye. When foods with gluten are eaten in people that are sensitive to gluten, they can cause an inflammatory effect in the body. The body works to counter the adverse effects that gluten can have on the body. Symptoms commonly experienced by people that are sensitive to gluten include stomach upset, headaches or bodily aches and pains.

The inflammatory response is especially true for people that have a medical diagnosis of Celiac Disease. To reduce internal harm from the effects of gluten, those with Celiac Disease need to practice strict avoidance when it comes to eating products that contain gluten. This can be found in many foods, so getting comfortable reading food labels, for this reason, is very important. Bread, muffins, bagels, pasta, rolls, cakes, cookies and crackers are just some of the foods that gluten can be found in. With the rise of attention made to gluten in the last few years, many companies clearly label their products if they are gluten-free, so they are easy to find.

More and more health professionals and physicians are speaking out about people that do not have Celiac Disease but are indeed gluten sensitive or have a true allergy to wheat. They are finding that some people still have problems with foods that contain gluten even with no diagnosis of Celiac Disease. Severe reactions can include hives, rash or anaphylactic shock, which requires immediate medical attention.

Alcohol

Initially, consuming alcoholic drinks induces feelings of relaxation, mild euphoria and happiness for many people. It can ease the worry or anxiety that a lot of people feel. This is only temporary. Depending on certain factors such as gender, weight and tolerance, alcohol and its effects can cause feelings of anxiety. For some people, this happens while they are drinking. Mood changes caused by alcohol can cause excessive worry, aggression and even anger. For others, when alcohol produces the 'hangover effect' the next morning, feelings of anxiety may accompany the hangover. The anxiety can vary in intensity from mild to severe. Alcohol also often leads to dehydration, with symptoms that can mimic anxiety.

Drugs

Recreational or illegal street drugs are a common contributor to anxiety and inflammation. A person may use these substances for social or entertainment purposes. Some people use these options to self-medicate to feel better in the attempt to escape from reality, relax and gain some peace of mind. As an example, some people use marijuana to try to decrease feelings of anxiety and it can be very effective. For others, marijuana use can cause or increase feelings of anxiety.

The worry about adverse side effects and other negative general effects on health from using drugs is also ample reason to cause worry and anxiety. Some of these drugs can cause a person to feel calm, at first. As the effects of a drug wear off and it leaves the bloodstream, the feelings of anxiety may increase. This is especially true for drugs that are addictive and that create a dependency. Sometimes the only way to decrease the anxiousness is to consume the substance regularly and in greater amounts.

Inflammation in the body arises from the negative or ill health effects that drugs can cause, depending on the way it is consumed. This can cause irritation or damage to the lungs, mouth, throat, stomach or other body systems. Some people acquire a sustained increase in blood pressure from the regular use of drugs.

Legal, everyday substances like tobacco and other forms of nicotine also cause a rise in blood pressure. This can make a person feel anxious until the effect of the nicotine wears off. It is recommended that these are best avoided altogether to prevent the long-term side effects that can occur and temporary feelings of anxiety.

Vitamins and Minerals to Help Reduce Inflammation and Anxiety

The quality and amount of nutrients in our diet can not only reduce inflammation but work in the body to improve our mental state. Eating a healthy diet that includes foods that will be listed and described below can certainly reduce feelings of anxiety for many people. The focus will primarily be on plant-based sources, although some nutrients can be gained by eating animal or dairy products. There are so many mental health benefits gained by eating a whole-food, plant-based diet.

By eating healthy, the complex interactions from many different vitamins and minerals in these foods work in a multitude of ways to calm the mind. Incorporating healthy foods into the diet throughout the day can act to help improve brain function, which will result in less anxiety.

Vitamins and minerals are vital nutrients that the mind and body need. They will be most effective if consumed in the diet as whole, fresh foods. It is more beneficial to get the vitamins and minerals in food form rather than just by supplementing with those can be found in pill form. They work in complex ways to help the mind and body function at an optimum level. More research is being done every day on how consuming whole foods, compared to supplements, work to benefit the body and mind.

Occasionally, and on the recommendation and prescription of a physician or dietician, we can get these vitamins and minerals from a supplemental pill or multi-vitamin. If a lab test shows the diet is inadequate in any area, supplementation may be necessary. Be sure to follow the recommended amounts prescribed by your healthcare professional. It is also important to purchase supplements from a reputable vitamin manufacturer, so you can ensure you are getting a high-quality product.

More supplementation is not always better. Some vitamins and minerals are not water-soluble so they are not excreted out of the body. They can even have adverse effects if too much is taken. Some supplements can accumulate in the body and could be toxic if large amounts are taken. On the other hand, if not enough of a supplement is taken, there may be no benefit gained for overall health and to help balance the mental state of mind.

Vitamin D

Ideally, everyone should get adequate Vitamin D from being outdoors in natural sunlight. A daily dose of adequate sunshine or other bright light exposure can increase the serotonin level in the brain. Vitamin D can also help the body absorb calcium for strong bones. There are very few sources of Vitamin D that come from food. Vitamin D is one nutrient that our bodies have the ability to create. Vitamin D production occurs when the skin has adequate sun exposure each day.

In reality, many northern climates are dark for most of the winter. Most people venture outside fully bundled up dressed in coats, hats, and gloves during the winter. A lot of people work indoors where there is inadequate exposure to sunlight or poor artificial lighting. Some people find they have inadequate Vitamin D levels. This can affect mood and energy levels. It can also contribute to feelings of anxiety. Sometimes, supplementing the diet with Vitamin D is the most effective way to treat Vitamin D deficiency. Your physician will know the adequate amount to prescribe to counteract the effects of colder climates.

B Complex Vitamins

The group of B vitamins is extremely vital for people dealing with stress and anxiety. There are certain B vitamins that are more helpful than others, but all work together in the body and central nervous system to help balance mood. Again, it is ideal to acquire vitamins and minerals from whole foods rather than just supplements. Here are some ideas to get B Vitamins incorporated into a healthy diet.

Vitamin B1 or Thiamine, as it is commonly known helps with nerve function and metabolism. It can be found in peas, legumes, nuts, and seeds. It is also found in whole grain foods like bread and flour.

Vitamin B2 or Riboflavin is also important for energy metabolism in the cells. It is primarily found in leafy green vegetables, other dark green vegetables, and whole-grain food products.

Vitamin B3 or Niacin is very important for balancing mood and in the transfer of energy between cells in the body. It is most often found in high-protein products such as nuts, seeds, legumes, avocado, and fortified whole-grain food products.

Vitamin B5 is also called Pantothenic acid. It helps to metabolize energy from the foods that are eaten. Good sources of Vitamin B5 include legumes and other whole-grain enriched food products.

Vitamin B6 is essential for the nervous system by aiding the neurotransmitters in the brain to function most efficiently. A reduction in anxiety is dependent on healthy neurotransmitter function. Great sources of Vitamin B6 come from potatoes, bananas, nuts, seeds, and beans.

Vitamin B7 or Biotin is also needed in the body for energy metabolism but in smaller amounts. It can be found in cauliflower, mushrooms, avocados, sweet potatoes and nuts.

Vitamin B9, also known as folate or folic acid is important in energy metabolism and for blood health. It is found in a wide array of foods such as oranges, avocado, asparagus, broccoli, brussel sprouts, green leaf lettuces, spinach, and peanuts. Folate can also be found in vitamin-enriched foods like crackers, bread, pasta, and breakfast cereals. Just make sure to read labels and choose whole grain, low sugar versions.

Vitamin B12 is unique in that it is primarily only found in animal products or attained in supplement form. Very few plant sources contain Vitamin B12 and in only very minimal amounts. Vitamin B12 is a type of bacteria or microorganism that animals get from the soil and then is passed on to humans who eat their meat. People on a whole-food, plant-based diet or other vegan or vegetarian diets need to take a Vitamin B12 supplement to get ample amounts. Your physician can recommend the best source or supplement and advise on the amount needed.

Choline is not technically a B vitamin but is a nutrient placed in the B vitamin complex group. It is also important for a healthy nervous system and neurotransmitter function and helps to balance and regulate mood. Rich sources come from beans, nuts, whole grains and vegetables such as shiitake mushrooms, red potatoes, broccoli, and cauliflower.

Other Vitamins and Minerals

Magnesium is a very important mineral that is required for optimal mind and body function. It plays a crucial role in the central nervous system to balance mood and keep anxiety at bay. Many common everyday stressors can deplete magnesium. Stress that originates from anxiety can deplete magnesium levels in the body. Magnesium can also be lower in people taking some pharmaceutical medications or are diagnosed with certain health conditions like heart disease and diabetes.

The body stores a small amount of magnesium, but it is still necessary to eat healthy to get adequate amounts. It is very important to eat a diet that contains magnesium-rich foods. A physician or dietician may recommend taking magnesium in supplement form when going through periods of high stress and anxiety. Dairy products and fortified foods contain magnesium. Some healthier ways to get magnesium are from eating a diet plentiful in green vegetables and lettuces, nuts, grains, and beans.

Potassium is a mineral that helps to counteract the effects of sodium in the diet. Having an adequate amount of potassium helps the body excrete sodium from the body when levels are high. Potassium is needed to help maintain normal blood pressure, heart rate, muscle, and nerve function. It plays a very important role in maintaining balance in the body to help reduce feelings of anxiety. Some foods to get potassium from include grapes, spinach, beans, and citrus fruits.

Omega-3 Fatty Acids support a healthy heart, reduce aches and pains and are vital for a well-functioning central nervous system. They work in the body to reduce inflammation and contribute to a more balanced mood. To lessen anxiety, the diet should include plentiful amounts of Omega-3 fatty acids. They are found in very high amounts in walnuts and ground flaxseeds. Other good sources include squash, green vegetables, and leafy greens and edamame (whole soybeans). Omega-3 fatty acids are also abundant in animal sources such as fatty fish like salmon, halibut, tuna, oysters and sardines.

Omega-6 fatty acids from plant sources can be beneficial for reducing anxiety. They should be included in minimal amounts to benefit healthy brain function. These include some plant and vegetable oils used for cooking and flavoring. Too much in the body can increase inflammation. Most people get too many omega-6 fatty acids from animal food sources which is detrimental. It is best to source these in the diet from plants, nuts, and seeds.

Vitamin K, eaten in adequate amounts in the diet may help reduce anxiety. It is an important nutrient to maintain healthy blood cell function and can play a role in keeping blood sugar balanced.

Zinc, selenium, and zeaxanthin are some trace minerals that come from a healthy diet that can decrease inflammation and anxiety. They also work as antioxidants in the body. They function to keep the cells of the body healthy by reducing or repairing the damage. Zinc also acts with insulin in the body to balance blood sugar. Whole grains contain selenium.

There are many essential amino acids required to aid normal body functioning. Nine of these amino acids are essential to maintain good health. Amino acids work to provide energy from the diet. They also help the body to heal and grow. A diet rich in vegetables, fruits, protein and fats (eaten in moderation) from plant sources can help our bodies use these amino acids most effectively.

As previously mentioned, probiotics are the 'good' bacteria that encourage and maintain good gut health and help to reduce inflammation. Probiotics can be taken in supplement form but are also found in fermented foods and drinks and in some dairy products.

Food and Drinks That Can Reduce Inflammation and Anxiety

Stay Hydrated   When in doubt, drink more water! Sometimes, one of the best things that a person can do to promote good health and reduce the feeling of anxiety is to keep hydrated. Generally, staying hydrated can result in better-looking skin, a normal functioning GI tract and feelings of well-being. Every single cell in the body functions most effectively when a person is fully hydrated. A person should be drinking an average of eight 8 ounce glasses of water per day. This amount should be varied depending on activity levels and the surrounding environment. For example, a person taking a hike on a hot day in direct sunlight will need to drink more water to be adequately hydrated.

Some people need to keep it interesting to drink enough water daily. A good way to encourage or stay motivated to drink water throughout the day is to flavor it. Fruit slices, like orange, lemon or grapefruit, can be added and makes drinking enough water every day more manageable. Some people like to add some cucumber slices to their drinking water.

For some people it is possible during the cooler months of the year, to keep a large bottle of water in the car. Keep reusable bottles of water in your bag, purse or backpack so good, clean water is always available for you to drink and refill easily.

Leafy Greens and Other Vegetables

Spinach, kale, arugula, and other dark, leafy green vegetables are full of nutrients like riboflavin, folate, potassium, and magnesium. Eating them will help reduce inflammation and stress in the mind and body.

Other varieties of greens to include in a healthy diet to reduce anxiety are swiss chard, rainbow chard, bok choy, mustard greens, beet greens, parsley, leeks, romaine, red leaf lettuce, and green leaf lettuce. Different varieties of sprouts such as broccoli sprouts, sunflower seed sprouts, bean sprouts, and alfalfa sprouts are full of B vitamins and essential amino acids, which is beneficial.

 For more adventurous tastes, green algae and seaweed are others that are high in these vital nutrients. They can be mixed into other foods like soups or casseroles or eaten alone, baked and seasoned.

There are so many high-nutrient vegetables in markets and grocery stores today that are readily available, affordable and worth eating to help reduce anxiety. Others not mentioned previously are tomatoes, which are high in potassium. Beets are also high in potassium and help to maintain healthy blood pressure. Potatoes, sweet potatoes, and yams are high in fiber, potassium, B vitamins. There are many other varieties such as white, gold, red, fingerling and the most common, russet. Green, red, orange and yellow bell peppers are a really good source of potassium. Hot peppers such as jalapenos, Anaheim, poblano and serrano contain many vitamins and are anti-inflammatory. Green and red cabbage, all the varieties of winter squash, celery, okra, parsnips, and garlic are all healthy items to add to the diet to help reduce inflammation and anxiety.

Fruit

There are many fresh and dried fruits to include in the diet which can help reduce anxiety. Eat those that are in season for the highest nutritional content and freshest flavor. Try to eat berries regularly for maximum antioxidant and anti-inflammatory benefits. These might include some of the more common varieties such as blueberries, raspberries, strawberries and raspberries and cherries. Due to local regions, there may be others that are grown in your area. Eat dried fruit such as raisins, dried cranberries, prunes, dates, dried apricots or tart cherries.

Other ideas for fruits high in vital nutrients to help reduce anxiety are bananas, kiwi fruit, apricots, pineapple, lemons, limes, oranges, cantaloupe, honeydew melon, and watermelon.

Nuts and Seeds

Nuts are a popular food to eat to help reduce anxiety because they are a rich source of protein, b vitamins, magnesium, potassium, omega-3 fatty acids, and essential amino acids. Each serving size is small so only a small handful is needed. Nuts are a good plant source for healthy fats so they should not be eaten in large amounts. Almonds, peanuts, walnuts, cashews, hazelnuts, pecans, pistachios, sunflower seeds, pumpkin seeds, brazil nuts are just some of the variety of nuts that can be included in a healthy diet to reduce anxiety.

Seeds contain high amounts of omega-3 fatty acids and Vitamin B6. Ground flaxseeds are very high in omega-3 fatty acids and are a reliable plant source. Make sure to eat ground flaxseed, not whole flaxseed. Our bodies are not equipped to break down the whole seed. Ground flaxseed can be mixed into oatmeal, smoothies and other recipes.

Chia seeds and chia sprouts are a great source of omega-3 fatty acids, magnesium, and zinc. Chia seeds are also a rich source of protein. These can also be mixed into smoothies, drinks, and other recipes.

Nut Butters

Peanut butter, almond butter, sunflower seed butter, and sesame butter are tasty choices that are good for us and keep inflammation down. They are very filling and provide high amounts of fiber and B vitamins. Nut butter can be very versatile in the diet. They can be eaten in sandwiches, on celery, with a banana, for making peanut sauce in savory dishes, etc.

Whole Grains

Quinoa and amaranth are two of the highest protein grains found in the world. They contain high amounts of fiber, potassium, magnesium and B complex vitamins. Oats, whole wheat, brown rice, bulger and barley, rye and popcorn are some other whole grains that are high in vitamins and minerals. They contain good amounts of fiber and have antioxidant properties.

Oatmeal

Try to eat oats in their more natural form. Steel-cut or other slow-cooking oats are less-processed, so withhold more nutrients and fiber. They have been shown to be healthier than the more processed, quick-cooking '2-minute' oatmeal.

Salmon and Tuna

As mentioned before, some fish that are higher in fat contain the beneficial omega-3 fatty acids that are helpful in lowering stress and anxiety. They also contain ample amounts of vitamin B6, vitamin B12, Niacin, potassium and Vitamin D.

Avocado

Adding avocado to the diet can have positive benefits to our brain and body. It is high in the B vitamins niacin and folate. It is also high in saturated fat so it should be eaten in moderation. Avocado can be spread on whole-grain or whole-wheat toast. Sliced raw avocado can easily be added to tacos, burritos, enchiladas, and other foods. Guacamole is a great way to add a lot of flavor to meals when made with cilantro, lime, onions, garlic, and tomatoes.

Beans and Lentils

These are very high in fiber, protein and B vitamins. There are so many choices and recipes for beans and lentils these days. Black beans, kidney beans, red lentils, green lentils, garbanzo beans (chickpeas), cannellini beans, great northern beans, lima beans, and soybeans are some great healthy options.

Buying beans already cooked in the can is an easy way to implement them into your diet. They are easily cooked into meals using a crockpot. Chili, soup, and stew are great ways to add beans to the diet. Eating hummus, made with chickpeas, with vegetables or on whole grain pita bread is a great way to get your daily protein in. Beans are very filling and can be a part of a main dish, instead of animal products. It is even more affordable to buy and use dried beans. Follow the directions to soak the beans properly and cook into your favorite meals and recipes.

Soy-Based Foods

Tofu, miso, edamame, soy milk, soy cheese, and roasted soy nuts are high in protein and Omega-3 fatty acids. Be sure to buy organic and non-GMO (genetically modified organism) soy products as these contain some of the highest amounts of pesticides and herbicides from certain farming techniques. The high amount of added chemicals may negate the positive benefits gained, so it is important to buy organic and non-GMO for this reason.

Fermented Foods

Fermented foods like pickles, pickled vegetables, sauerkraut, kimchi, miso, and tempeh have been found to encourage gut health and reduce overall body inflammation. Yogurt and Kefir are also considered fermented foods. When purchasing these foods, be sure to find brands that don't have artificial colors or refined sweeteners in the ingredients list. Most natural health food stores carry these types of fermented foods in the refrigerated section.

Kimchi is a fermented vegetable dish that can be purchased or made at home. Traditionally, it is eaten as a Korean side dish. Today many people include kimchi in their diet as a snack or included in a meal. There are many easy 'How To' recipes online that can be followed. Kimchi usually consists of largely chopped Napa cabbage or bok choy, daikon radishes, green onions, leeks, dried red peppers, ginger, some form of sugar, soy sauce and fish sauce (optional). Kimchi can be mild to spicy and can include other vegetables, depending on preferences.

Miso is a fermented soybean paste. It can also be made from other grains, barley or rice. It is commonly used as a seasoning in Japanese foods. Many people all around the world eat miso for its health benefits. It can be used for making soup but can also be used to make sauces, rubs, marinades and salad dressings. The lighter-colored miso has a milder flavor while the darker miso pastes have a stronger flavor. The reason the miso will be used for and what the flavor preference is, will determine what type of miso to use.

Tempeh is a fermented soy product traditionally eaten in Indonesia. It is a fairly well-known food in natural health food circles. Tempeh is easily used as a meat substitute where more texture is desired (versus tofu). It can be used in place of dishes that traditionally use meat. It is high in calcium and other vitamins and minerals. Tempeh is versatile because it can take on a variety of other flavors in dishes like stir-fry, stews, soups but still retains a meat-like texture and shape.

Kombucha is a fermented drink that is beneficial and comes in many flavors that people enjoy. Many restaurants and stores make this drink and it can be bought in a single serving or bulk sizes to go.

Drinks to Help Calm Anxiety

There are many drinks available to buy or make that are having calming properties. These include green tea, chamomile tea, lemon balm tea, pomegranate juice, passionflower tea, lavender tea, valerian root tea, kava tea, blueberry lemonade, and raspberry lemonade, to name a few.

Herbs and Spices

Food should never be boring! Healthy food should taste good, look good and use high-quality ingredients. Adding some herbs or spices can give a bold kick to healthy foods. Being able to enjoy the food you eat is so important for sticking to a lifestyle that is good for you and your brain. As an added bonus, many herbs and spices are known for their anti-inflammatory properties. Some of these powerful, flavorful spices include turmeric, ginger, parsley, black pepper, cumin, coriander, chili powder, paprika, cinnamon, and clove.

Dark Chocolate

Cocoa can provide enjoyment and health benefits as well as reduce anxiety. Different chocolates contain different amounts of dark chocolate. Aim for the healthier versions that have less refined sugar and higher amounts of dark chocolate. Read the label for information on chocolate content and choose those with a higher percentage. In addition to reducing anxiety, chocolate is an antioxidant. Eating more is not always better. The high amounts of sugar, fat, and calories that come from eating chocolate can negate some of the benefits. Enjoy this food but eat in moderation!

Healthy Food Ideas

The meal choices below are just some suggestions to get started eating a healthy diet to reduce inflammation and lower anxiety.

Breakfast Options

- One serving of oatmeal (usually ½ cup to ¾ cup) with ¼ cup of blueberries, glass of almond, cashew or soy milk

- Whole wheat pancakes or waffles, with brown rice syrup, real maple syrup or agave syrup; ½ cup sliced strawberries

- Sweet Potato or Potato Veggie Browns – slice or chop thin, add onions, green bell pepper, chopped kale, tomatoes, and turmeric or curry seasoning. Cook in a small amount of olive oil, add water to lightly coat; cover and steam for 10 minutes to finish cooking through. Optional for a big weekend breakfast: Top with a cooked egg and/or cheese, sprouts, salsa or hot sauce.

- ½ cup low-sugar granola with almond, cashew or soy milk; top with raisins or dried cranberries or other fresh fruit (blueberries, strawberries, banana slices, peaches).

Lunch Options

- Turkey (or other plant-based meat replacement) sandwich on whole wheat bread or in whole wheat or veggie tortilla with lettuce and tomato (can add mustard, onions, pickles, cucumbers, sprouts, etc.). Use mayonnaise sparingly. Half an orange, sliced up.

- Veggie Option: hummus in a whole wheat pita or tortilla. Add cucumbers, red onions, greek olives, tomato and sprouts or spinach.

- Sliced Veggies with hummus – red, orange, yellow or green bell peppers, broccoli, cauliflower.
- Steamed artichoke with non-dairy butter or vegan mayo.
- Baked Potato with chopped vegetables for toppings.

Dinner Options

- Baked Salmon (with lemon, garlic, rosemary). Baked potato with butter and sour cream. Large spinach or kale Salad (top with chopped or sliced vegetables like tomatoes, artichoke hearts, bell peppers, sweet peppers).
- Taco Salad – taco-seasoned chicken (for plant-based option, use kidney beans or black beans), romaine lettuce, tomatoes, green onions, olives, avocado, cilantro, salsa, organic corn tortilla chips or baked tortilla slices.

Dessert Ideas

- Baked pears or apples with small amount of butter and brown sugar
- Homemade apple or peach crisp
- Raspberry or strawberry rhubarb crisp

Healthier Options for Condiments and Sauces

- Ketchup made with real cane sugar (no high fructose corn syrup)
- Salsa, red sauce, Verde sauce
- BBQ sauce (no high fructose corn syrup or other 'natural flavors')

- Vegan or vegetarian mayonnaise or garlic aioli (plant-based)
- Organic mustard
- Salad dressings - Balsamic (buy from the store or use your own balsamic vinegar, olive oil, minced garlic, fresh lemon, and salt and pepper, to taste); vegetarian or vegan salad dressings (no milk, eggs)
- Non-dairy sour cream
- Non-dairy butter

Day 1

Breakfast: 1 cup whole grain, low sugar cereal with ¾ cup milk; ½ cup strawberries

Snack: 15 pretzels with 2 tablespoons hummus

Lunch: Spinach salad with 3 cups fresh spinach, 2 tablespoons pumpkin seeds, 3 sliced mushrooms, 6 cherry tomatoes, 5 croutons, and 2 tablespoons salad dressing

Dinner: 3-4 ounces grilled chicken breast with 2 tablespoons BBQ sauce served with ½ cup brown rice and 1 ½ cups steamed broccoli

Dessert or snack: 1 banana with 2 tablespoons almond or peanut butter

Day 2

Breakfast: ½ cup oatmeal made with 1 cup milk; add 2 tablespoons dried cranberries, 1 tablespoon brown sugar or honey

Snack: 1 sliced orange bell pepper, 2 tablespoons hummus

Lunch: 2 cups Potato Chickpea Curry, one apple

Snack: High protein, low sugar granola bar

Dinner: Taco Chicken Salad (use taco or fajita seasoned baked chicken breast, chopped or shred; 3 cups chopped lettuce, chopped tomatoes, sliced black olives, green onions, ½ cup shredded sharp cheddar, salsa or hot sauce, dollop of sour cream)

Dessert or snack: 2 tablespoons dark chocolate almonds

Day 3

Breakfast: Wheat whole or whole-grain toast with 2 tablespoons avocado, 1/4 cup chopped cucumbers, ¼ cup chopped tomatoes, top with sprouts and no-salt seasoning; banana

Snack: Banana with 2 tablespoons almond butter

Lunch: 2 cups Layered Cornbread Salad, 1 apple

Snack: 1 cup baked beet chips with 2 tablespoons hummus

Dinner: 3-4 ounces baked, seasoned salmon, ½ cup brown rice, 2 cups steamed broccoli with butter

Dessert or snack: 1 medium homemade oatmeal cookie

Day 4

Breakfast: ½ cup steel cut oats, 1 cup almond or cashew milk with 1 tablespoon honey and ¼ cup blueberries

Snack: ¾ cup celery sticks, 2 tablespoons vegan cream cheese, 2 tablespoons raisins

Lunch: 1 medium baked potato, 2 tablespoons butter, ¼ cup shredded cheese, melted; chopped, lightly cooked vegetables, such as broccoli, onions, tomatoes, mushrooms for topping; ¼ cup sour cream

Snack: ½ cup raspberries

Dinner: Black Bean Sweet Potato Enchiladas served with guacamole; small side salad with 1 tablespoon salad dressing

Dessert or snack: Frozen fruit bar

Day 5

Breakfast: 2 frozen whole wheat or whole grain instant waffles, 3 tablespoons maple syrup, 2 vegan sausage links

Snack: one apple

Lunch: 2 cups Quinoa Salad

Snack: 1 cup broccoli dipped in ranch dressing

Dinner: 2 cups Chicken and Wild Rice soup, 2 cups dark green leafy salad with tomatoes, cucumbers, a few croutons and dressing

Dessert or snack: 1 cup fresh, sliced pineapple chunks

Day 6

Breakfast: Veggie browns (sliced or cubed potato, ½ bell pepper, ¼ cup chopped onions, ¼ cup mushrooms, etc.) – saute in 1 tablespoon olive oil, cover to steam until done, add salt, pepper, and other seasonings; mix in an egg to cook

Snack: Orange

Lunch: 3 cups spinach salad with chopped vegetables, 2 tablespoons salad dressing

Snack: 2 tablespoons cashews

Dinner: 2 cups Broccoli Tofu Stir Fry, ½ cup brown rice

Dessert or Snack: Apple Crumble

Day 7

Breakfast: 2 eggs, cooked how you prefer; 2 pieces whole-wheat or whole-grain toast with 2 tablespoons margarine; 1 sliced kiwi fruit

Snack: 1 serving baked pitas with 2 tablespoons spinach dip

Lunch: almond butter and whole fruit jam sandwich;

Snack: ½ cup cherry tomatoes, ½ cup snap peas, 2 tablespoons greek yogurt-based spinach dip

Dinner: Portobello cheeseburgers, 1-2 cups oven-baked potato fries or sweet potato fries, seasoned to taste

Dessert or snack: ½ fresh mango, sliced

'Healthier' Recipe Ideas

Quinoa Salad

This is one of our family favorites due to some members of our family being on a whole-food, plant-based diet. This can be made with no dairy or animal products. This salad can be eaten as a quick lunch, side dish or due to the high protein content of quinoa is great as a light dinner during hot summer months. It has also been a favorite at potlucks for those who have more adventurous and healthy preferences.

To reduce the sodium content in this recipe, boil the quinoa in water instead of the vegetable or chicken broth. The Greek olives and saltiness of the feta cheese (if you decide to use it), usually provides plenty of salt. You will need a large salad bowl to serve it in.

Ingredients:

4 cups vegetable or chicken broth

2 cups dry quinoa

1 cup chopped red bell pepper

½ cup chopped green onion

½ cup sliced Greek olives

½ cup diced red onion

1 cup sliced cherry tomatoes OR 1 chopped red Roma tomato

1 can artichoke hearts, chopped

2-4 ounces crumbled feta cheese (depending on how salty the quinoa cooked in broth turns out; omit if making the salad vegan)

1/3 cup cilantro, optional

1/3 cup parsley, optional

Dressing:

¼ cup fresh squeezed lemon juice

¼ cup red wine vinegar

3 teaspoons minced garlic

2 tablespoons olive oil

Black pepper to taste

Directions:

Bring quinoa to boil in vegetable or chicken broth.

Cover and reduce heat to low to simmer.

Cook for 15-18 minutes or until all liquid is absorbed.

Chop the vegetables while quinoa is cooking.

Set cooked quinoa aside to cool.

While quinoa cools, make a dressing combining all ingredients.

Combine veggies in a large salad bowl.

Stir in cooled quinoa and feta cheese.

Top with dressing and mix.

Serve at room temperature or chilled.

Black Bean Sweet Potato Enchiladas

This is another family-friendly recipe that is very filling and can be adapted to whatever tastes and dietary needs there are. For the youngest family member, I try not to make this too spicy. For added spice, each of us can add hot sauce or locally-made salsa to each serving. One large stovetop cooking skillet and one 9x13 rectangular baking dish needed.

Ingredients:

1 package corn, wheat or whole grain tortillas (any size)

1 tablespoon olive or avocado oil

1-2 tablespoons taco seasoning

1 cubed yam or sweet potato

1 cup finely chopped kale

½ chopped red or yellow onion

1 can black beans, drained

1 can diced tomatoes (can use fresh, when available)

1 large can green or red enchilada sauce

1 can sliced black olives

1 small can diced green chiles

2 cups shredded sharp cheddar (can be non-dairy)

Sliced avocado, optional

Chopped fresh cilantro, optional

2 tablespoons sour cream, optional (can be non-dairy)

Hot sauce, optional

Fresh salsa, optional

Directions:

Put olive oil, onions and sweet potatoes in a skillet on low to medium heat.

When skillet is hot and vegetables are starting to cook, add ½ cup water, taco seasoning and kale to pan. Mix well.

Cover and steam for 10-15 minutes or until sweet potatoes are slightly tender when pierced with a fork. If there is still a lot of water in a skillet, simmer on low with the lid off to evaporate the remaining liquid.

Add tomatoes and black beans. Stir together well.

Preheat oven to 350 degrees.

Start laying out tortillas to fill. Add ½ to ¾ cup vegetable black bean mixture from skillet into each tortilla (can do one at a time if space is limited).

Disperse mixture evenly to use up all the tortillas. As you fill them, roll them up and put them in the pan. If using 12 large tortillas they can be arranged in pan tightly.

Pour enchilada sauce evenly over all enchiladas. Top with green chiles.

Bake uncovered 45 minutes to 1 hour (or when enchilada sauce starts to bubble). In the last 5-10 minutes, sprinkle shredded cheese on enchiladas. Let melt completely.

Take out of the oven and let sit for about 5 minutes. Add black olives and diced green chiles.

Cut into desired serving sizes (will make approximately 8 servings). Top with cilantro, salsa, hot sauce, sour cream, avocado.

Easy Guacamole

Ingredients:

2 avocados, ½ cup of your favorite salsa, garlic salt, to taste and fresh juice

of lemon or lime.

Directions:

Cut avocado in half. With a spoon, scoop avocado seed out. With a knife, cut

vertical and horizontal lines into each half. Scoop out avocado chunks into a bowl. Add salsa, a sprinkle of garlic salt and a fresh squeeze of lemon or lime

into the bowl. Mix well and enjoy with tortilla chips.

Chicken and Wild Rice Soup

This is another family favorite for cold, winter days. It is a hearty, filling soup. I have made this as is, or by omitting the meat and dairy products and substituting plant-based products for a vegan version. Both work equally well, although they taste a little different. You will need to precook wild rice and chicken breasts and will need a large soup pot.

Ingredients:

1 stick butter

2 tablespoons minced onion

½ cup flour

3 cups chicken or vegetable broth

2 cups cooked wild rice (cook this ahead of time)

½ cup chopped carrots

½ teaspoon salt

2 cups cooked chopped chicken breast (boil to cook ahead of time; can be shredded)

1 can evaporated milk (or use non-dairy milk)

Chopped chives, optional

Chopped or slivered almonds, optional

Directions:

Melt butter in a pot on low to medium heat. Saute onion in melted butter.

Blend in flour, stirring as you add. Add broth slowly while mixing until smooth.

Keep stirring and increase the heat until the mixture comes to a boil, for 1 to 2 minutes.

Decrease heat and add the cooked rice and chicken, carrots, salt, and milk. Simmer on low for 5-10 minutes.

Serve while hot. Garnish with chives and almonds, optional.

Potato Chickpea Curry

My whole family enjoys a flavorful curry dish. This recipe is quick for busy weeknights. Other vegetables can be added for more nutrients and texture. Sometimes it can get too spicy, but that is easily fixed with extra coconut milk or some plain greek yogurt.

Ingredients:

2 medium russet potatoes

1 tablespoon olive or avocado oil

½ white or yellow onion, chopped

2 minced garlic cloves

2 teaspoons cumin

1 teaspoon cayenne

5 teaspoons curry seasoning mix

1 teaspoon salt

½ teaspoon pepper

1 bay leaf

1 teaspoon finely chopped fresh ginger

1 chopped red, yellow or orange bell pepper

1 can diced tomatoes

1 can chickpeas

1 can coconut milk

1 package frozen peas

1 small container plain greek yogurt

Small Naan flatbread, optional

Directions:

Clean and chop russet potatoes into bite-sized cubes. Boil until tender when pierced with a fork (about 10-15 minutes). Drain and set aside.

In a large soup pot, heat oil on low to medium heat. Add onions and garlic. Stir until cooked thoroughly.

Add cumin, cayenne, curry, ginger, salt, and pepper. Mix well.

Add tomatoes, chickpeas, peas, bay leaf, and boiled potatoes. Mix well. Simmer for 10 minutes. Serve hot. Add a dollop of Greek yogurt to tame flavor if too spicy. Eat with Naan.

Broccoli Tofu Stir Fry

Our family loves a good, easy stir fry for a quick weeknight dinner. The main ingredients can be as varied as what is available in the refrigerator. It just takes a little imagination to make it delicious. You will need a small cooking pot and a large skillet.

Ingredients:

1 cup uncooked brown rice

2 heads fresh broccoli

2 cloves minced garlic

1 tablespoon chopped ginger

1 package firm tofu

4 tablespoons olive or avocado oil

1 tablespoon rice vinegar

1/3 chopped onion

1 chopped bell pepper

1 package sliced mushrooms

½ cup vegetable broth

½ cup of soy sauce

3 tablespoons honey

1 tablespoon sesame oil

Optional: ½ cup teriyaki sauce

Directions:

Put 2 cups water and 1 cup brown rice in a small pot and bring to a boil. Cover, put heat on low and simmer approximately 45 minutes (or follow directions on package).

Take the tofu out of the package, pat dry with towels. Put in colander, place a heavy object on tofu and set in the sink (to draw out water). Let sit for 15 minutes.

Wash and chop the remaining vegetables. Cut broccoli heads off stalks and break up with hands or cut into single pieces.

In a large skillet, turn the heat on low. Add olive oil. Take the tofu out of the colander and neatly slice into bite-size squares.

Put tofu in the skillet, turn heat up to medium and keep turning to lightly brown on all sides (will be golden in color). Make sure there is adequate oil to keep the tofu from sticking to the pan, but not too much. When browned, set aside in a bowl.

In skillet, place broccoli and vegetable broth. Cover and steam on low for 10 minutes.

Add onions, garlic, ginger, bell peppers, and mushrooms. Increase heat to medium to cook. You may need to cover for a few minutes to make sure all is cooked evenly.

Add soy sauce, rice vinegar, honey and sesame oil (other option to use in place of these ingredients - use a good quality teriyaki sauce, that isn't made with high fructose corn syrup). Mix well.

Lightly fold in cooked tofu pieces and heat thoroughly.

When all is cooked, serve over rice.

Layered Cornbread Taco Salad

This is an old family favorite. It is tasty and includes a good mix of vegetables and is completely filling on its own – no side dishes needed. This is another good one for friends and family get-togethers and potlucks. This could be made vegan, but this current recipe I use is not (includes eggs and dairy). You will need a very large serving bowl or salad bowl.

Ingredients:

1 box Jiffy cornbread mix (or other quick baking mix)

1 can corn, no salt, and no sugar

1 can beans (your choice of kidney beans, pinto beans or black beans)

1 orange or yellow chopped bell pepper

1 large Roma tomato, chopped

2-3 bunches Romaine lettuce, chopped

1 can sliced black olives

½ bunch green onions, chopped

1-2 cups shredded sharp cheddar

Dressing:

1 cup sour cream

1 cup mayonnaise

2-3 Tablespoons Taco Seasoning

Make the dressing by combining all three ingredients. Let sit until time to add to the layered salad. (For a lighter dressing, use plant-based mayonnaise and sour cream. Amounts can be decreased to ¾ cup each.)

Directions:

Cook cornbread mix, according to directions in a small bread loaf pan. Let cool thoroughly, to room temperature, while you chop remaining vegetables.

Once the bread is cool, cut or crumble bread into a large salad bowl. Distribute evenly.

Drain and rinse beans. Drain corn. Pour beans over cornbread crumbles. Pour corn over beans. Put chopped bell peppers over corn. Make sure to layer evenly.

The largest layer will be the chopped romaine lettuce. Put this over the bell peppers.

Dollop the dressing lightly over romaine. With a spoon, spread the dressing in an even layer over the lettuce.

Add 1-2 cups of shredded cheese overdressing layer. Top with roma tomatoes, black olives, and green onions.

Homemade French Fries

Ingredients:

4-6 Russet potatoes or sweet potatoes, washed well and cut into strips

Seasonings of your choice – No-Salt Seasoning, Seasoned Salt, Garlic Salt, etc.

2-3 Tablespoons Olive Oil or Avocado Oil

Directions:

Preheat oven to 350 degrees.

Place potato strips on a baking sheet.

Drizzle olive or avocado oil on top. Lightly mix into potatoes.

Bake for 45 minutes or until cooked through, tender and lightly browned.

Serve with ketchup, ranch or homemade fry sauce.

Portobello Burger

For those people that enjoy mushrooms, this is a tasty, juicy alternative to a regular hamburger. It is very filling and all of the same toppings can be used as on a hamburger. They cook quickly on a BBQ or stovetop and can even be baked in the oven.

Ingredients:

Large Portobello mushrooms washed with stems removed

Brie or Swiss cheese

Olive or Avocado Oil

Seasoning or salt

Burger ingredients of your choice – whole wheat or whole grain hamburger buns, romaine lettuce or fresh spinach, sliced tomatoes, sliced onions, pickles, ketchup, mustard, mayonnaise

Directions:

Lightly brush mushroom with oil on both sides

Place in a warmed stovetop skillet or on a hot grill. Season, if preferred.

Cook on each side for a few minutes, until mushroom is tender and cooked through. If using cheese, put cheese on to melt.

Apple Crumble

I have been making this dessert for about 20 years and the whole family loves it. The ingredients change depending on what fruit is in season. This recipe is very easy to make. You'll need a round baking pan or an 8x8 pan will do.

Ingredients:

5 cups chopped fresh fruit (apples or rhubarb, whole raspberries or any combination of other fruit)

¾ cup flour

½ to 1 cup sugar (depending on how sweet the fruit is)

½ teaspoon cinnamon

½ teaspoon salt

¼ lb butter, in small pieces (or softened in microwave)

Directions:

Preheat oven to 350 degrees.

Place chopped fresh fruit in a pan (you may have to use more fruit depending on the size of the pan). Fill with fruit until almost full.

In a separate bowl, combine flour, sugar, cinnamon, and salt.

Add softened butter to mix until it resembles coarse crumbs (if you use a lot more fruit, you may want to double the crumble ingredients because that's the best part).

If the mix seems to wet, slowly add flour and sugar until it crumbles.

Spread crumble mix lightly and evenly over fruit (don't worry if the crumble mix seems stacked too high; the fruit will sink down as it bakes).

Bake for about 1 hour or until crumble is lightly browned.

Option: serve with ice cream (there are many soy, coconut and other plant-based options available).

Here is hoping your journey to lessening or eliminating anxiety is a successful one! There are so many options to eat healthy to reduce inflammation in the body. It takes patience and a willingness to learn and try new things. When a healthy lifestyle can be maintained for the long-term, you will start to see results in many areas of your life, not just in mental health.

One last thing!

I want to give you a **one-in-two-hundred chance** to win a **$200.00 Amazon Gift card** as a thank-you for reading this book.

All I ask is that you give me some feedback, so I can improve this or my next book :)

Your opinion is *super valuable* to me. It will only take a minute of your time to let me know what you like and what you didn't like about this book. The hardest part is deciding how to spend the two hundred dollars! Just follow this link.

http://reviewers.win/anxietydiet